# Fast Metabolism Diet
## Fast Weight Loss

By Cathy Wilson

Copyright © 2014

Copyright © 2014 by Cathy Wilson

ISBN-13:
978-1503256583

ISBN-10:
1503256588

All Rights Reserved. No part of this publication may be reproduced in any form or by any means, including scanning, photocopying, or otherwise without prior written permission of the copyright holder.

First Printing, 2014

Printed in the United States of America

## Income Disclaimer

This book contains business strategies, marketing methods and other business advice that, regardless of my own results and experience, may not produce the same results (or any results) for you. I make absolutely no guarantee, expressed or implied, that by following the advice below you will make any money or improve current profits, as there are several factors and variables that come into play regarding any given business.

Primarily, results will depend on the nature of the product or business model, the conditions of the marketplace, the experience of the individual, and situations and elements that are beyond your control.

As with any business endeavor, you assume all risk related to investment and money based on your own discretion and at your own potential expense.

## Liability Disclaimer

By reading this book, you assume all risks associated with using the advice given below, with a full understanding that you, solely, are responsible for anything that may occur as a result of putting this information into action in any way, and regardless of your interpretation of the advice.

You further agree that our company cannot be held responsible in any way for the success or failure of your business as a result of the information presented in this book. It is your responsibility to conduct your own due diligence regarding the safe and successful operation of your business if you intend to apply any of our information in any way to your business operations.

## Terms of Use

You are given a non-transferable, "personal use" license to this book. You cannot distribute it or share it with other individuals.

Also, there are no resale rights or private label rights granted when purchasing this book. In other words, it's for your own personal use only.

# Fast Metabolism Diet
## Fast Weight Loss

By Cathy Wilson

# Table of Contents

Introduction .................................................................. 9
Metabolism Explained ................................................ 13
Factors Affecting Metabolism Rate ....................... 17
Scientific Evidence - The Science of It ................. 23
Tips and Tricks to Improve Your Metabolism ..... 27
Fast Metabolism Diet Overview ............................ 39
Myths/Truths Metabolically Speaking .................. 47
All about Food and the Fast Metabolism Diet
Concept ................................................................. 53
Sample Life Tips to Sustain Your Hard Efforts .... 65
Final Thoughts ..................................................... 69

# Introduction

Did you know that without metabolism you couldn't possibly exist? Your body wouldn't have the physical ability to burn energy or generate heat to keep you agile and functional.

**The metabolic energy burning process is seriously important!**

Common sense says that understanding and utilizing this natural and mechanical ability of the body, is a useful tool to maximize fat burn, slim you down to sexy, and sustain the results.

*Journal Advocate* states weight management is really mathematical. You simply balance the number of calories you ingest, against the number of calories you expend. If you know the number of calories used, you can figure out how many calories your body needs to gain or lose weight.

**Logically simple on paper. Not so easy in real life!**

Before exploring this exciting discovery of encouraging the body to work harder for you in order to burn more energy faster, I want to make it clear this in an **introductory** or **investigative** book.

By no means is this *"The Metabolism Diet Book Bible,"* written for all PhD graduates, specializing in Biochemistry and Kinesiology, and related *EXPERT* fields.

I write with a deep knowledge but to an introductory audience. People looking to get their feet wet and utilize scientifically proven simplistic measures to lose weight and get healthy long-term!

What's important is positive perspective. Zeroing in on the basic facts, and engaging your mind, body, and soul to gain practical useful information to create **your** master wellness plan.

A diverse and ever-changing eating, exercise, and positive lifestyle strategy to blast fat for good!

**NEWSFLASH!** *There is no one diet that works for everybody.*

More than likely there's not a single diet plan that **always** works for any one person – not without making continual changes in the base game plan.

And this Fast Metabolism Diet concept isn't **PERFECT** either!

It's a fantabulous eating concept **INTRODUCING** you to healthy eating strategies. A book that **WILL** better you as a whole if you're open to it.

**BRIGHT LIGHT OF LOGIC** - You owe it to your good health and wellness to open your thoughts to gather strategies, concepts, tips and tricks, from a variety of weight loss diet plans, and create a unified original strategy for you.

To be effective you'll have to make changes to it regularly. Tuning attentively to what your body is telling you. Making sure you're armed mentally to override a lot of what your head is saying.

Let's face it, we're creatures of habit with oodles of habits that really suck.

There's always room for improvement right?

It's time for a positive changes. Ones you'll grow to enjoy and eventually transform into healthy habits for life. This will help you maintain your weight comfortably at the set point of your choosing. Enabling you to make minor adjustments easily and swiftly as time marches on, and the natural life cycle plays out.

You are unique. So are your body and mind. And your chosen method of fueling your body should be too!

The Fast Metabolism Diet is just one logical eating plan that makes sense. Apply what works considering your tolerance and preferences, and you're one gynormous step closer to your primary health and wellness goals.

**Ready...Set...Go!**

# Metabolism Explained

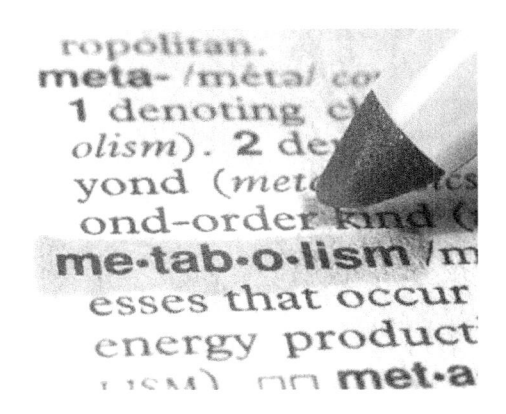

## What is Metabolism?

It's a term derived from Greek, which basically means *to transform or change*. The processes that occur within your internal systems can be defined as a set of chemical and physical changes within the body which produce energy to support life and create new materials. This process could also be measured in terms of how the body converts various foods into energy, and at what pace it uses this energy. That's if you have your science cap on.

The process of metabolism is triggered when the absorption of vital life nutrients commences. That seems simple enough!

*Science Daily* defines metabolism as the biochemical process of combining vital nutrients with oxygen to release the energy your body requires to function.

**Your Basal Metabolic Rate or BMR** measures the amount of energy or calories required just to maintain your body weight at rest. Your BMR is responsible for approximately 75 percent of the energy you burn each day.

**Metabolism Units are made from nutrients and include:**

***Amino Acids** - from proteins such as lean beef
***Fatty Acids** - from fats i.e. butter
***Glucose** - from carbohydrates mainly derived from whole grains

**Metabolism Purpose**

If you didn't have a metabolism you wouldn't be able to burn food for energy in order to function physically. You literally and figuratively wouldn't have the energy to roll over, hit the snooze button, and head back to Dreamland. Or give your partner an early morning snuggle!

**Metabolic Phases**

*Last I heard there were just two!*

***Catabolism**** - Process that decomposes the tissues to generate the energy your body requires to function properly.

***Anabolism**** - Creates reserves, new cells, and maintains your body cells constructively. The result is the generation of skin tissues, nerves, and muscles.

Hormones like thyroxin help regulate metabolic activity whether catabolic or anabolic. Just after you've munched down a healthy grill chicken salad with lime zest, anabolic activity is in full swing.

On the flip side, when you're sweating buckets at the gym it's the catabolic activity that hogs the limelight.

**Next we'll take a quick peek into the dominant metabolic processes, which are:**

***Digestion**** -- Where *food* is the material that enables energy to create new tissues and store it as fat for later use.

***Circulation of Blood**** - - Where the compounds are carried through the blood to the major organs set to use them.

***Body Heat Regulation**** -- Metabolic energy creates heat that helps regulate internal body temperature.

***Ridding the Body of** Waste (sweating, breathing, elimination) - These catabolic metabolic processes break down harmful toxins, creating waste the body gets rid of through the lungs, bowels, skin, and kidneys.

By understanding the process and purpose of metabolism your mind is better equipped to comprehend how and why the **Fast Metabolism Diet** concept is valuable in getting control of your weight and well-being.

*My Thoughts...*

*Your metabolism is extremely important for your overall good health. It provides the energy your body relies on to run, jump, dance and sing.*

*Internally this energy is used for breathing, cell repair, and other essential bodily functions. You need energy for every single thing you do, and without metabolism your time is up!*

*Poor metabolism can lead to serious health issues like diabetes. Where your body is unable to process or metabolize sugar. This is a signal of the ultimate breakdown of your body.*

*By eating healthy, exercising, and living a healthy lifestyle you're going to ensure optimal metabolic function.*

*Let's look a little deeper into possible scenarios that help your metabolism work better for you.*

# Factors Affecting Metabolism Rate

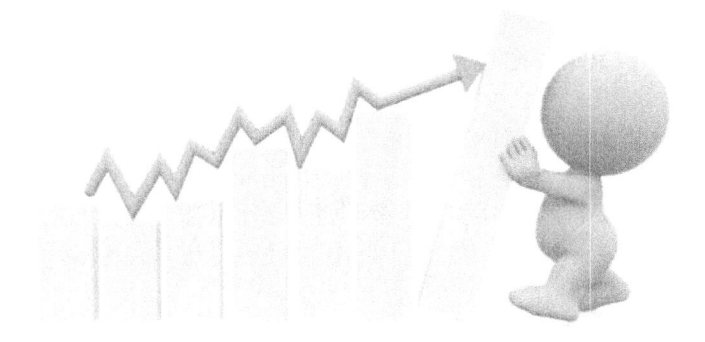

If your metabolism were solid, secure, and unbreakable, you'd be in deep trouble. Stuck exactly where you are without being able to gain, drop, or change your body composition at all. Luckily for all of us there are numerous variable factors affecting the rate at which your body burns calories.

**GAINING WEIGHT** -

If you gain weight you're naturally burning more calories because of an increase in size. If you gain muscle instead of fat you're ahead of the game because on a level-playing field muscle utilizes more energy than fat.

This makes muscle-building a brilliant move when looking to whip yourself into fantabulous shape!

**YOUR BODY SIZE** -

It makes perfect sense a larger body's going to have more cells that need fueling in comparison to a smaller body. If you're bigger in size your metabolism is *usually* higher than someone with a smaller figure.

**GENDER** -

This is one of those uncontrollable factors beneficial to gents only. Guys normally have more lean body mass than women. Scientists link this to the hormone testosterone, which of course is more abundant in males normally!

**YOUR BODY COMPOSITION** -

Your muscle-to-fat ratio determines your body composition. If you're flabby like the Stay Puff Marshmallow Man, then you're essentially loaded with fat. Fit and slim people with lots of lean muscle have a body composition that naturally has a higher metabolic rate compared to their out-of-shape twin, given similar circumstance.

**Makes sense to hit the gym doesn't it!**

**GENETIC MAKEUP -**

Another uncontrollable factor is your heritage or genetic makeup, according to experts at *Nutrition Today*. Genes will influence your metabolic efficiency. Explaining why people with pretty much the same weight, height, and body composition, burn energy at different rates.

**AGE -**

This is where the tick-tock of your life clock becomes a pain in the rear. Scientific research shows after the age of 30 it's natural for your lean body mass to reduce gradually, making room for fatty tissues...

*The result is slower metabolism.*

Experts mainly blame it on hormonal fluctuations.

**CHIN UP! ALL ISN'T LOST**

By following a stronger exercise regimen, and working hard to boost your lean muscle mass, you can counteract or rather battle this inevitable life change.

**It's your choice.**

Put in the time and effort and you can have an absolutely lean and beautiful body until death do you part.

### MENTAL STATUS -

This one gets a little bit complicated. When you're stressed and anxious your system's on high alert. This triggers more fat and calories to be used. Energy stores are broken down for these processes according to *Science Daily*.

However, many people that have issues with their mental capacity go way overboard on junk eating. So the tiniest increase in metabolic rate means diddly-squat against all the fat invading the tissues from constant overeating.

### HORMONES -

Most of your internal processes are regulated and controlled by hormones. By exercising regularly and increasing the rate key hormones are produced you're going to naturally increase your metabolic rate.

### SET BODY TEMPERATURE -

What's your body's physiological response to being chilled to the bone?

You shiver, right?

Shivering is the way your internal system tries to boost your body temperature by breaking down fatty tissues.

This is very much like increasing your natural body temperature through exercise. Shivering does the same thing because when your internal systems are working harder more fat and calories are required.

**NUTRITION HABITS -**

When, how much, and what foods you choose to eat all affect your metabolism.

Most of us overeat and stress out our system. This plays havoc with hormones and forces your body to become completely inefficient in maximizing the consumption of fat and calories you provide for energy.

**There's nothing to argue here.**

It's exactly why you see so many grossly overweight people pigging out like it was their last supper.

Keep in mind these key factors can directly change the rate at which your body naturally burns calories.

*My Thoughts...*

*You can't make informed decisions in life without knowing all the facts. Understanding the factors that affect your energy consumption rate helps you make the best metabolic decisions for yourself. It's best to have a look at the controllable here and just accept and live with the uncontrollable.*

*Unless of course you want to drive yourself nuts!*

*Changes can be made to your metabolism but only if you commit to it and have reasonable expectations.*

# Scientific Evidence - The Science of It

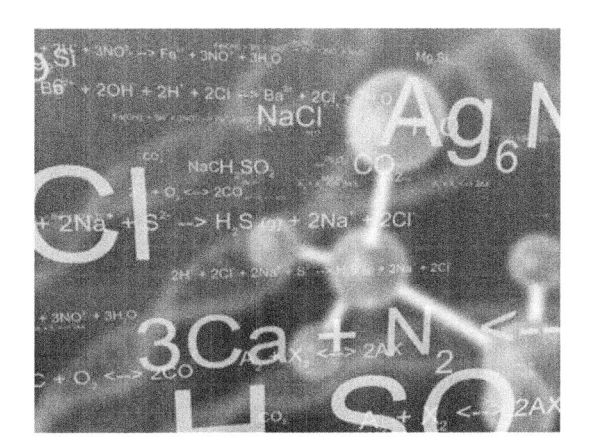

Don't fret, I'm not going all techno-statistical here. That's not what this book is about. However, a dash of science does seem to capture attention and serve up credit.

**FACT** - By boosting your BMR you're going to set your weight loss plans into motion.

In order to lose fat science says you need to take less energy in and use more energy doing it.

People are resistant to change as a whole. So when it comes to dieting or tweaking your eating habits, your resistance shoots straight through the roof.

This dieting concept has been around for quite some time and is the choice celebrities flock to when they need to get energized, lean, and sexy strong fast.

Celebs can be real quick about it since they're at a huge advantage in the disposable income department compared to *normal* folk.

Science also says by increasing the consumption of lean protein in proper amounts, and by exercising, you'll trigger your system to burn fat and build lean muscles, which also increases your metabolic rate.

So if you're building sexy, lean, and beautiful muscle, you'll burn more calories even when you're napping, compared to sitting on your lazy butt watching horror flicks with your flub.

Let's dig a little deeper into the nerdy science stuff.

### Scientific Pointers

*One pound of muscle burns about 14 calories per day. Whereas a pound of fat burns about nine. Sensibly, if you want to work with your body you should look to build lean muscle, particularly if you want to zap your rolls fast!

*Countless smarty-pants researchers report caffeine increases metabolism by boosting your heart rate. According to a report on ehow.com, your metabolism is increased about 10 percent with caffeine. Naturally women break down and absorb caffeine faster than guys do.

*As mentioned previously, it takes more energy to break down protein than fat. So by eating more lean protein in place of fat you'll kick your natural metabolism in the rear.

Scientists take the physiological makeup of the human body, and through experimentation under controlled conditions, measure various factors, deducing how the metabolism reacts.

Understanding what your body is made of, how the constituents utilize energy and what influences them, gives you the information required to maximize energy burn through metabolic adjustments.

Metabolism works just like a furnace. And although scientists can't explain everything, *most* of what they say makes sense.

*My Thoughts...*

*Having full confidence in the basic concept of an eating strategy is imperative. The Fast Metabolism Diet concept has the science necessary for people to open their minds and expect great results.*

***It's a definitive step in the right direction.***

# Tips and Tricks to Improve Your Metabolism

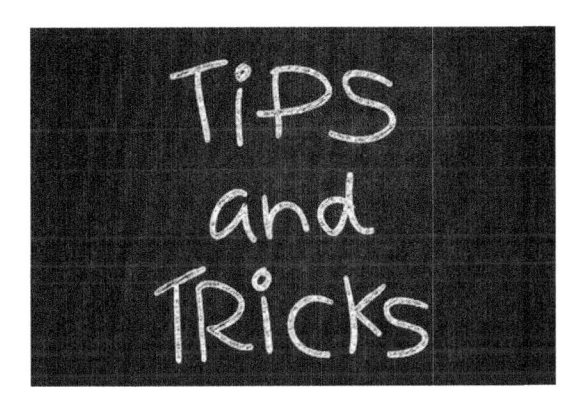

If you're looking to increase your metabolism you've got to open your mind to change. This means if you're just going through the motions hoping there's some secret button hidden somewhere that's going to eat your fat away, you're sorely mistaken.

It doesn't matter what sort of tactics you use to lose weight. They are **ALL** going to require constant effort and focus which is very difficult to sustain.

It's your initial changes in habit that's the first tough pill to swallow. The next is making minor adjustments regularly to ensure results are continuous. Leaving the final difficulty as finding changes you can turn into habit, and set them in stone for the long-term.

It's easy to see you've definitely got your work cut out for you. If you're up to the challenge, and understand that sitting on the couch munching on salty snacks isn't going to get you any slimmer, sexier, and more importantly healthier, then read on, and get happy knowing you're headed in **YOUR** right direction.

## EAT WHAT YOUR BODY NEEDS!

This is a tough one. Figuring out what amount of energy your body needs and making sure you aren't overfeeding, or under nourishing it, is freakin hard. What many people don't realize is eating too little is more restrictive and damaging than eating too much of the right thing.

Most people are programmed to believe in the paradox, the less food you eat the more weight you'll lose.

## THIS IS ALL WRONG!

If you aren't providing your body with enough energy to function it'll shut down on you, according to the nutritionists at *The University of Waterloo*. You're forcing your body slip into emergency mode and conserve.

**RESULT** - Every single thing you eat, no matter how minuscule, will be hoarded and stored as fat. Your metabolism will slow because your body is working against you, trying to use as little energy as physiologically possible.

The message here is mixed. Your body doesn't understand you're trying to lose weight.

By not giving it enough food you're communicating there's an emergency and right now your body needs to kick into survival mode, or you're eventually going to die.

Extreme but very true!

In caveman days this is what the body did as a defense to natural disasters, when there was no food to be found. Under these tragic circumstances even when the body slowed, starvation was often inevitable.

You have to eat *healthy* calories if you want to lose weight!

**SWITCH IT UP FASTING**

Studies show by changing your routine from time to time you'll boost your metabolism. Experts from *Science Daily* agree, fasting for a day, maybe once a month, is a good way to force your body to increase its metabolism naturally. A little bit of deprivation in moderation **WILL** help renew your furnace strength.

Understand also, more is not better.

If you fast too often your hormones and internal burning mechanisms will go haywire, and your body won't know up from down. By the time you signal to your body to start expending more energy it will have already halted the process.

**INGEST HEALTHY FATS**

**FACT** - Without fat you'd be dead.

The natural food breakdown process requires fat, preferably healthy or unsaturated fats in small doses. Natural fats help to regulate hormones and contribute positively in the fat breakdown process.

2-3 servings of healthy fats per day should suffice!

***Here are a few examples of healthy fats to add to your everyday meals:***

*Avocado
*Coconut, sunflower, and olive oils

*Olives
*Nuts
*Peanut butter (1tbsp)
*Non-hydrogenated margarine
*Fatty fish
*Flaxseed

**These healthy fats also help to:**

*Slow and prevent blood clots
*Lower triglycerides or *bad* blood fats that are directly associated with cardiovascular diseases
*Lower the chances of suffering from a stroke

*Moderation is key.*

Too much unsaturated fat in your diet is just as damaging as eating the wrong kind. Unhealthy saturated fats are found in deep fried dishes, butter, lard, and high-fat pastries.

## ADD A SERVING OR TWO OF LEAN PROTEIN

Your body uses lean protein to build lean muscle. The thermogenic effect comes into play here and indicates your body must work harder if protein is the nutrient of choice.

Generally 2-3 servings of lean protein are adequate each day for optimal function, according to *US Food and Drug.* If you happen to be weight-training your lean protein intake should increase.

Eggs, nuts, peanut butter, lean beef, chicken, and fish, are excellent sources. There's even adequate amounts of protein in milk, cheese, and yogurt. But one should be careful with these milk products, particularly with yogurt, cuz they're often sweetened with loads of sugar.

## MUSCLE BUILDING

By piling on the muscle through regular strength-training you'll significantly boost metabolism. Transforming your body into to a finely tuned fat zapping machine!

### *Supporting Facts...*

*The body does require more calories to fuel muscles than it does for melting pesky old cottage cheese fat.

*It's pretty simple. Build sexy strong muscles and send more fat packing. So if you want to lose fat there's **GYNORMOUS** potential in building up muscles.

*The more muscle you develop the greater your fat burning rate.

It's important to think straight here. Developing five pounds of muscle doesn't mean you're going to burn an extra 500 calories a day!

At best you'd expend an extra 70-75 calories.

Knowing you've gotta burn an extra 3,500 calories per day to shed just one pound of fat is what you need to focus on. Bottom line is, muscle building helps boost fat blasting, but is just one piece to the puzzle. It takes time and commitment to make it happen.

**BOOST FIBER INTAKE**

Many people trying to shed fat don't consider the importance of adequate dietary fiber, in optimal metabolic function. Fiber helps to level blood sugars, which is directly linked to your metabolism. Whole grains, fruits, and vegetables, are excellent sources of fiber.

*Did You Know?*

Your body doesn't have the enzymes required to break down fiber. So it goes straight out of your body, dragging toxins and waste with it.

*So Why Do People Tend To Gain Weight More Readily With Age?*

Without getting too technical in this beginner's book, it's got to do with blood sugar and insulin. Regulated or healthy blood sugar levels are necessary in the weight loss and the sustaining process.

As you age your blood sugar levels rise, making it very difficult for insulin to continue transferring sugar out of the blood and into the cells. LPL or lipoprotein lipase is the enzyme produced when insulin levels are escalating. Both LPL and insulin encourage fat cells to get fatter.

**Bottom line?**

Higher blood sugar levels cause increased weight gain naturally within the body.

All of this is interconnected with fiber, fat loss, and metabolism.

When blood sugar levels are high they're pushed further still when fewer calories are being eaten, in combination with high carbohydrates and low fiber.

So many *FAD* diets out there promote *VERY* low calorie eating, and are pumped full in the carbohydrate department. To make matters worse, fiber is seldom mentioned here.

These are a few very suspicious factors behind the miserable failure of fad diets!

Overseas experts report increased fiber assists with blood sugar control in diabetics. Studies also show fiber lowers bad cholesterol. Both point to the fact high-fiber eating makes sense for smooth systemic function and shedding layers.

**Fiber also assists in weight loss and control by:**

*Lowering insulin, and sending excess sugar out the door through the intestine

*Assisting with insulin receptor sensitivity, diverting sugar to fuel the muscles instead of fat

*Slowing sugar release, leveling out insulin production, and maximizing vitamin absorption

*Helping decrease bad cholesterol, Free Fatty Acids or FFA, and the circulation of harmful fats in the bloodstream

**TRAIN LEGS IN PARTICULAR**

Your Gluteus Maximus is the largest muscle in your body but your Rectus Femoris (legs) are also major players. Your quadriceps are muscles that run from the bottom of your hip flexor on the front of your leg, down to the top of your knee.

You'll feel the burn if you happen to be executing wall squats, or leg presses.

Since it's one of the larger muscles strength-training helps boost your metabolism. Involving more muscles in the exercising, sends the message loud and clear that more energy needs to be burned.

**RESULT** - This means you're losing more fat when you eat and exercising sensibly.

**AVOID OR LIMIT ALCOHOL**

Alcohol is loaded with calories that have zero value nutritionally. Alcohol has to be metabolized. This means it becomes priority one over any and all other internal breakdown processes. It's sent straight to the liver where oxidization takes place.

*Problems...*

Alcohol interferes with your body absorbing the nutrients it requires. Causing a gassy bloating that buggers up the functioning of your natural hormones.

Alcohol greatly influences your metabolic rate and ability to lose weight.

With alcohol you inhibit your body from making glucose. This eventually develops into glucose intolerance, often associated with diabetes and weight gain.

Saving your alcohol for special occasions makes both your metabolism and fat loss plans happy!

**EXERCISE REGULARLY**

Exercising regularly temporarily increases your metabolism. The more often you exercise the greater calories your metabolism burns. Even when finished exercising your body still burns calories at a higher rate for up to 72 hours afterwards, according to exercise specialists at *Men's Fitness*.

**STOP SMOKING**

Don't think I really need to be telling you to stop smoking. There's not one single thing good about it.

Smoking forces poisonous toxins into your body, slowly but surely killing you. One major issue is smoking deprives your organs of getting the oxygen they need to thrive. Without adequate amounts of that gas, how is your body going to optimize the metabolic process?

Your body works like a finely tuned instrument and interfering knowingly has consequences.

**PICK UP PACE!**

Another trick to kick that metabolism of yours up a few notches is to pick up pace during your regular day.

***Without putting in a lot of effort you can...***

- *Park a few blocks away from work so you can walk

- *Choose stairs over the elevator

- *Run to get the mail instead of walking leisurely

- *Hustle up the stairs at home instead of climbing them normally

- *Walk instead of sitting in the park

- *Stretch the moment you step out of bed to get the juices flowing

- *Walk instead of riding in the golf cart

- *Take the family to the park instead of watching television

- *Go for a power-walk during lunch break

- *Cut the grass with a push-mower instead of a sit-down

You get the idea.

*My Thoughts...*

*Every little bit helps. By figuring out simple strategies to boost your metabolism you're only going to speed up the weight-loss process.*

*As humans we're creatures of habit, resistant to change. Good or bad we like doing the same things over repeatedly and hate the idea of different.*

*Mind over matter.*

*Decide first you want to make changes. Then use these tidbits of advice to make a real difference.*

# Fast Metabolism Diet Overview

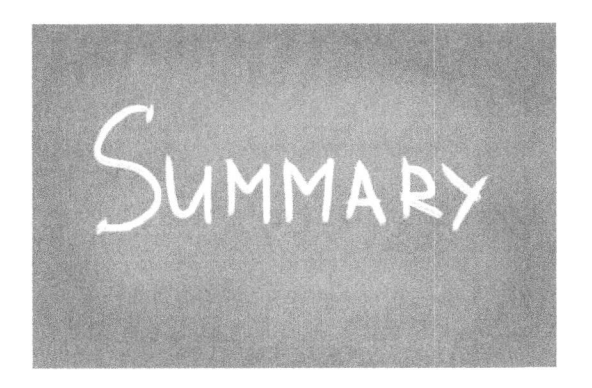

The "Fast Metabolism Diet" concept is widespread. It's used by oodles of nutrition and health experts, including the well-known health and wellness consultant, *Haylie Pomroy*.

Each specialist has a slightly different view from their peers on the Fast Metabolism Diet concept.

**CONSENSUS** - Their personal interpretations show how best to tap into your natural metabolic processes to zap fat and get healthy.

**MAIN BELIEF...**

Simply put, fat-burning power foods help shed pounds off your frame in record time. Eat more food and lose weight sounds pretty good to me!

Some success stories using this eating strategy claim to have shed up to 20 pounds in just one month. Using food as a nutritious means to encourage your body to lose weight makes perfect sense.

**CIP - Cathy's Important Point** - The rate in which people burn metabolize fat is different. However, it's critical to set realistic expectations in weight loss. According to *Scientific America*, it's physiologically impossible to lose more than 2-3 pounds per week safely and long-term.

Aiming for 1-2 pounds with smarter eating choices and regular exercising is your **BEST** move.

This diet or eating plan encourages you to eat healthy, nutritious, and beneficial foods more frequently. Preferably mini-meals every 2-3 hours if you can. This triggers increased thermogenic activity because you're teaching your body to trust it will constantly have fuel. This encourages your metabolism to kick into high gear.

The idea, which is similar to intensive interval training at the gym, is to keep your body and metabolism guessing.

Like most diets the Fast Metabolism Diet is broken down into phases.

**Phase 1**

This phase is called **Carbohydrates** and takes place on days one and two. The idea with this primary phase is to prepare your body to get thin and beautiful.

This is much like giving a child a toy when preparing them to clean their room!

Healthy and complex carbohydrates, including whole grains and fruits, are on the menu. The benefits you enjoy are both mental and physical. Vitamins and minerals trigger *feel good* endorphin release, with the intention of boosting your mood and eliminating harmful cravings.

Carbohydrates also encourage the release of hormones T3 and T4, which speed up your metabolism.

**Phase 2**

Here we shift into the **Protein and Vegetable phase**. The focus for days three and four, is getting plenty of lean protein. Mainly from meats and fish, along with nutrient-and fiber-rich tasty vegetables.

This phase communicates to your body it's time to start kicking fat rolls right out the door. Your hormones start listening. Working harder to melt fat for good.

The protein is excellent for supporting growth of new lean muscle tissue, which helps increase your metabolism further, burning more fat in the process.

**FACT** - Even at rest, a muscular body burns more fat than a flabby one.

By ingesting low-sugar foods, you're naturally signaling to your soon-to-be sexier body, fat storage isn't cool. These foods help your body get the message loud and clear, that you don't want fat accumulation. Sending your body signals to work harder.

This also messages to your body to sweat harder than it does, when you plant your lazy butt on the couch, and munch away on the junkiest junk you can find!

*Stop acting like you don't know what I'm talking about!*

Low-sugar foods also strengthen your adrenal glands, and streamline the flow of digestive enzymes. This helps your body work for you, not against.

**Phase 3**

Here, we shift into oils and healthy fat on days five, six, and seven of this eating plan. Some call it the light at the end of the tunnel, where your metabolism gets very happy eating those healthy fats found in oils, avocado, fish, and nuts.

**Now you're physically and mentally set to lose fat.**

Bringing your cleverly stored fat out into the open where it can be burned off as fuel, is exactly what you want. The focus is on your thyroid gland and the T4 hormone which it readily manufactures.

T3 can singularly take your body's ability to melt fat to a whole new level. The fats are utilized as fuel to work your body. They're located in the mitochondria, which are the brains of each cell, according to *Tech World*.

The goal is to signal to your body to continuously create more T3 through the trigger of hormones. All of which happens when more *healthy fats* are consumed.

Fatty fish like salmon, nuts, and avocado, are great sources to start with.

To this fat incinerating process you'll add lean meat and veggies. Choline and inositol are key nutrients for burning fat and transporting cholesterol to the liver.

Choline is also required to form the neurotransmitter acetylcholine, which helps ensure optimal functioning of the peripheral and central nervous systems. It's found in foods like liver, wheat germ, salmon, and shrimp.

Inositol is present in the outer layer of your cell membranes, helping with the normal functioning of your nervous system and making sure that messages get through.

Both choline and inositol are naturally found in the body. Soybeans, oranges, and other citrus fruits, wheat germ, nuts, and whole grains, contain inositol. Be sure to get your fair share of Phase 3 of the Fast Metabolic Diet.

For your eating strategy you'll want to eat the healthy fats we've already mentioned. Also, ensure you get three eating sessions per day with medium amounts of lean protein and good carbs. Two snacks should include two healthy fats of your choice; half an avocado and 1/4 cup of walnuts, for example.

**\*This fast metabolism eating strategy concept is all about cycling nutrients.**

It's a trick your body can't detect reports the experts at *Weight Watchers*. Always seeming to have the nutrients it requires readily available encourages your body to naturally boost your metabolism, and zap fat consistently. Faster than it normally would if programmed to know exactly what you're eating, when, and how much.

The idea with this strategy is **NOT** to count calories, but focus on the foods in each phase.

Make sure you pay attention to your bodily hunger cues and it won't take long for results.

Increase success by knowing exactly how much food you need to eat to lose a particular amount of weight. You can adjust and readjust according to your wants, needs, desires, and personal weight loss goals.

**You are in the driver's seat here!**

By sticking with this eating plan you'll teach your body to trust you, increase your metabolism rate, and burn your fat stores off fast and effectively.

With this diet you don't need to worry about forcing your body into *starvation mode*, where it protectively lowers your metabolism and starts to store anything and everything you eat as fat.

**A simple intrinsic human survival mechanism.**

Your system will get plenty of essential vitamins and minerals it requires to thrive under this Fast Metabolism Diet concept.

Now you've got the information required to take action! As unique as you are this concept is the solid platform you can build the weight loss program that works for you.

*My Thoughts...*

*The Fast Metabolism Diet concept truly makes great sense when just discussing nutrition. The idea of diversity and change is beneficial,*

*especially when you're looking to drop weight and keep it off.*

*This forces your mind and body to keep guessing and burn optimal calories consistently!*

# Myths/Truths Metabolically Speaking

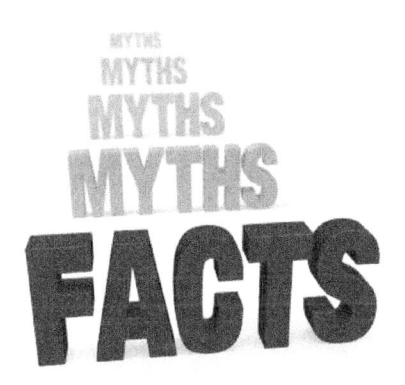

When it comes to long-term fat loss the metabolism gets the short end of the stick!

**THE CLAIM?**

***"Oh well, I've got slow metabolism and that's why I am always going to have thunder thighs."***

On the flip side, when someone's skinnier than a stick bug, people automatically assume they've got an eating disorder, or are just *gifted* with a super-fast metabolic rate.

Think of your body as a huge fire to heat your house. The food you consume is the same as the logs you'll toss into the fire to feed it. The metabolism is the rate at which the fire burns these logs to keep your house toasty warm.

Depending on the size of your fireplace you may need more or less logs than your neighbor does.

Your metabolism is the amount of calories required each day to satisfy your basic energy needs. This means breathing, cell growth and maintenance, circulation, temperature control, and any other need that's essential for survival.

These basic energy requirements make up about 75 percent of the total calories you burn each day according to *Dr. Jan Moreau*, MD, Barrie, Ontario. On that note, it's time to set straight a few misconceptions about your metabolism.

**MYTH ONE**

**Most skinny people are just born with a fast metabolism rate.**

**THE TRUTH**

Sure your BMR is created from your genetic makeup, sex, age, weight, and height to begin with. But the relationship between how much you weigh and your metabolism isn't what you might think.

According to *FitMetabolism* founder *Jason Hagen*, who lives in Canada, *"A smaller person may naturally burn fewer calories per day, whereas an obese person burns more calories."*

Essentially the BMR measures the energy you need to maintain basic function, which in turns makes it logical that a larger person requires and burns more calories.

Just think about this for a minute. Let's assume a 6 foot, 250 pound overweight man, and a 5 foot 7 inch, 110 pound woman, have been lying in bed for a month straight.

Both are eating the high-fat, 4000-calorie diet of the obese man. You can pretty much guarantee the skinny woman with a so-called fast metabolism rate is going to get fat!

If the plan were flipped and the overweight man consumed the measly 1,500 calories a day the skinny woman uses for fuel he'd surely drop a few pounds at some point.

That just makes sense.

**MYTH TWO**

**When you hit the age of 40 your metabolism slows noticeably and every year after that it declines at an alarming rate.**

**THE TRUTH**

WOW! When did this person get off the turnip truck? Oh, that's just so wrong! Sure, as you age your body slows and starts to break down. And if you sit on your rump and accept muscle and bone breakdown, wrinkling, more creaks and cracks, and all the other nuisances of aging, then yes, you're not going to burn off that Christmas dinner quite so quickly.

*IS THIS INEVITABLE?*

NO!

By taking a stand to eat healthier and take extra special care to work your body hard to build lean muscle mass, improve strength, agility, flexibility, and mobility, through exercising and strength-training, you can kick this myth in the rear and actually fire up your metabolism for all the right reasons.

**MYTH THREE**

**Eating spicy foods burns loads more fat.**

**TRUTH**

Now wouldn't that be nice! Yes, spicy hot foods do cause a slight increase in temperature, meaning a slight increase in the rate at which you burn calories. But experts agree it's not enough to beat suffer the consequences of breaking out the extra hot sauce. Sorry about that. So opting for the fiery hot chicken wings over the sweet and succulent honey garlic isn't going to cut it.

## MYTH FOUR

**Whacky hormones make people fat and there's really nothing they can do about it.**

## THE TRUTH

Your thyroid function directly reflects the running of your BMR; meaning if your thyroid isn't pulling its weight you may burn fewer calories. The opposite is true if your thyroid is trying to be *Speedy Gonzales*.

However, these conditions are incredibly rare and easily detected and treated. If this is your reality then get the diagnosis and put a treatment plan in place.

Hormones are essential in *normal* metabolic function. They respond to exercise.

No matter what stage of life you're in exercising will deter metabolic slumps, not to mention boost your mood, as if you've taken a handful or two of happy pills!

## MYTH FIVE

**You can handle a slower metabolism rate by eating less and not bothering with breakfast most days.**

## THE TRUTH

Are you nuts! Talk about totally messing up your body and head! If you periodically and unpredictably starve your poor self, what do you think it's going to do?

First of all your body won't trust you. This means when you desperately want to shed fat stores it's just going to hoard and store them as much as possible.

It'll also lower your metabolism, slow digestion, and make fat stores last longer.

**SMART MOVE!** Eat regular well-balanced meals and stop messing up your metabolism.

These are a few myths that clearly steer people in the wrong direction, away from their skinny jeans and into their Velcro fat pants.

*My Thoughts...*

*There's always gotta be someone spreading rumors that screw everybody else up. By finding the truths about metabolism you can take and use this information to blast that pesky fat, and put a beautiful smile upon your face.*

# All about Food and the Fast Metabolism Diet Concept

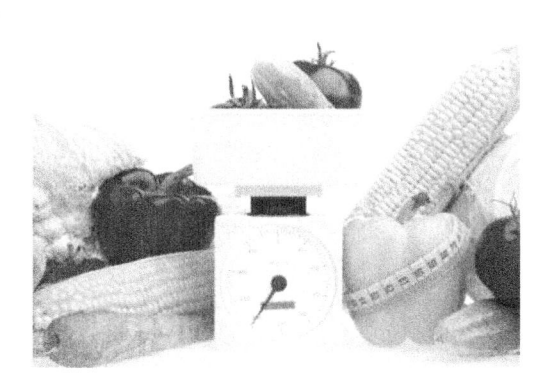

This is the chapter you don't want to miss. It's loaded with information on what you should be eating with each phase, why, and how much. Along with understanding what **no-no foods** to avoid.

There's also info on grub-related strategies too. These tidbits will help you understand what

Action steps need to be taken so you're able to take action fast and **GET RESULTS!**

**PHASE 1** (Days 1-2)

In Phase 1 you want to eat **THREE** meals consisting of good-carb, medium protein, and low-fat foods, plus **TWO** fruit snacks each day, eating every 3-4 hours.

**Sample Outline of Day**

*Breakfast* -- Fruit and grain immediately

*Snack* - Fruit 3-4 hours later

*Lunch* -- Vegetables, fruit, protein, grain, 3-4 hours later

*Snack* -- Fruit, 3-4 hours later

*Dinner* -- Protein, grain, veggie, 3-4 hours later

**Proportion Sizes Standard**

*Lean Protein* -- 6 ounces of fish, 4-5 ounces lean meat or 1/2 cup legumes all phases

*Veggies* -- No limit with phase appropriate choices

***Grains*** -- 1/2 cup pretzels or about a cup of cooked grains

***Fruit*** -- One piece

***Eggs*** -- 3-4 egg whites

***Fat*** -- Don't add any

**Possible Food Options**

***Veggies*** -

*Mixed Greens
*Eggplant
*Carrots
*Celery
*Green Onions
*Beans
*Chiles
*Kale
*Leeks
*Lettuce
*Arugula
*Mushrooms
*Onions
*Parsnip
*Peas
*Arrowroot
*Peppers
*Pumpkin
*Rutabaga
*Spinach
*Broccoli
*Sprouts
*Spirulina

*Yams
*Tomatoes
*Cabbage
*Squash
*Turnips
*Zucchini
*Bamboo Shoots
*Cucumbers

*Fruits* -

*Apples
*Any Berry
*Pears
*Cantaloupe
*Figs
*Grapefruit
*Melon
*Kiwis
*Limes
*Mango
*Guava
*Kumquats
*Lemons
*Oranges
*Papaya
*Peaches
*Pineapple
*Tangerines
*Watermelon

*Protein* -

**\*Lean Red Meat** - -Pork, buffalo, beef
**\*Lean Poultry** -- Chicken, game, turkey, fowl

***Processed -deli meats that are nitrate-free*** - Corned beef, sausage
**\*Lean Fish**
**\*Egg White Only**
**\*Beans**

*Other* -

**\*Herbs** -- All
**\*Spices** -- All
**\*Sweeteners** -- Stevia or Truvia
**\*Grains/Starches** -- Brown rice, barley, amaranth, brown rice pasta, buckwheat, Kamut (Khorasan wheat), millet, steel-cut oats, quinoa, spelt, sprouted grain, wild rice
**\*All Nut Flours**
**\*Brown Rice Milk**
**\*Brown Rice Cheese**
**\*Tapioca**
**\*Water, Herbal Tea**

**PHASE 2** - (Days 3-4)

Here you're looking to get started with the fat blasting process! You want to eat **THREE** high-protein, good-carb, low-fat meals, **TWO** protein snacks, eating every 3-4 hours.

**Sample Outline of Day**

*Breakfast* -- Protein and veggie right away

*Snack* -- Protein

*Lunch* -- Veggie and protein choice

*Snack* -- Protein

*Dinner* -- Veggie and protein

**Proportion Sizes Standard**

*Lean Protein* - Same as Phase 1

*Veggies* - Any amount of qualified vegetables

*Egg Whites* - 3-4

*Fruits* -- Same as Phase 1 with approved fruits, eat **LOTS** of green ones, low sugar, alkalizing

**Possible Food Options**

*Veggies* -

*Arugula, Asparagus, Beans, Cabbage, Broccoli, Celery, Cucumbers, Fennel, Endive, Chiles, Onions, Leeks, Kale, Lettuce (no iceberg variety), Mixed Greens, Peppers, Mushrooms, Watercress, Swiss Chard, Spinach, Rhubarb, Shallots

*Fruits* -

*Lemons, Limes

*Lean Protein* -

***Lean Red Meat** - Beef, buffalo, wild game, pork

***Lean Poultry** -- Chicken, turkey

***Processed Meats** -- Same as Phase 1

***Lean Fish** -- Same as Phase 1

***Shellfish**

***Egg Whites**

*Other* -- Same as Phase 1

**Foods to Avoid Phase 2**

*****Starchy Vegetables*** -- Like bamboo shoots, carrots, potatoes, tomatoes, peas, pumpkin

****No Fruit*** -- Except lemons and limes

****No Sugary Salsa and Ketchup***

****No Fats, No Nuts, No Seeds***

**PHASE 3** - (Days 5, 6, 7)

Now it's time to get burning fat seriously! Eat a medium amount of good-carbs, lots of healthy fat, low-sugar fruits, and a medium amount of lean protein, thyroid triggering foods.

Each day look to have **THREE** meals and **TWO** snacks, with 2 fruit, 4 fat/protein, 5 veggie, and possibly 1 grain.

This phase makes sure you get enough healthy fat each day. Choose higher fat protein options to help.

## Sample Outline of Day

***Breakfast*** -- Fruit, fat/protein, grain, veggie, right away

***Snack*** -- Veggie, protein/fat

***Lunch*** -- Fruit, veggie, protein/fat

***Snack*** -- Protein/fat, veggie

***Dinner*** -- Veggie, fat/protein, grain if you want

## Proportion Sizes Standard

***Veggies*** -- As many as you want if on phase list

***Protein*** -- Same as Phase 2

***Eggs*** -- 1 normal egg

***Grains*** -- 15 grams crackers or half cup cooked

***Fruits*** -- Same as Phase 2

***FAT*** -- 1/4 cup nuts, 1/2 avocado, 2tbsp nut butter, 3-4 tbsp. dressing

## Possible Food Options

### Veggies -

*Same as Phase 1

### Fruits -

*Same as Phase 1 **PLUS** coconut products, including milk

### Lean Meats -

*Same as Phase 1

### Fish -

*Same as Phase 1

### Eggs -

*Whole

### Other -

*Legumes, nuts, seeds

*All beans

*Nut milk

*Barley, oats, quinoa, sprouted grain

*Nut flours

*Brown rice produces

*Broths and condiments

*All* herbs and spices

**Healthy Fats -**

*Avocado*

*Nuts*

*Seeds*

*Oils*

*Hummus*

Drink LOTS of water!

**Basic Rules of Eating**

It's recommended you start this eating concept on a Monday so you can stick easier with the work schedule of the corporate world. With the typical work week from Monday through Friday, weekends are left for exploring, and possibly *treating* yourself.

Of course you choose what works for you.

**Here are a few more pointers to keep you on the straight and narrow**!

*If you're looking to blast a heck of a lot of fat you should eat more healthy food in general. This helps keep your metabolism elevated and ready for serious action.

This sample food outline concurs with looking to drop under 20 pounds.

**Foods to Avoid**

Here, we'll take a look at foods that aren't helpful in boosting your metabolism.

**If you're optimizing this fast metabolism eating concept it's recommended you stay clear of the following foods:**

***WHEAT** -- Such as crackers, breads, pastries, cookies, rolls

You can have sprouted wheat.

***CORN** -- This includes all corn products, corn, tortilla chips, cornstarch, and corn cereals

***DAIRY** -- This means no yogurt, milk, cheese, butter, no *low-fat*!

***SOY** -- The only exceptions are Bragg Liquid Aminos, and Tamari

***REFINED WHITE SUGAR** -- Even a few teaspoons will interfere with weight loss

***CAFFEINE** -- This includes decaf

***ALCOHOL**

***DRIED FRUIT**

*FRUIT JUICES

*ARTIFICIAL SWEETENERS -- Exceptions are Stevia or Truvia

*FAT-FREE -- Just stay away from this!

My Thoughts...

Having a plan of action for anything you do is important. Understanding when you should be eating, how much and what, is critical to your fat-loss success.

Think of it as the meat and potatoes of this eating concept, minus the potatoes, unless they're sweet!

Beware you may have to do a little fine-tuning, depending on your general food knowledge, preferences, and weight loss goals.

Don't expect to be perfect. Just do your best, allow for mistakes, and adjust when required.

If you're unsure of something don't just guess. Ask a qualified professional to remove the guesswork from the equation. Believe in yourself and take action.

You may trip and fall for a while but you **WILL** get results!

# Sample Life Tips to Sustain Your Hard Efforts

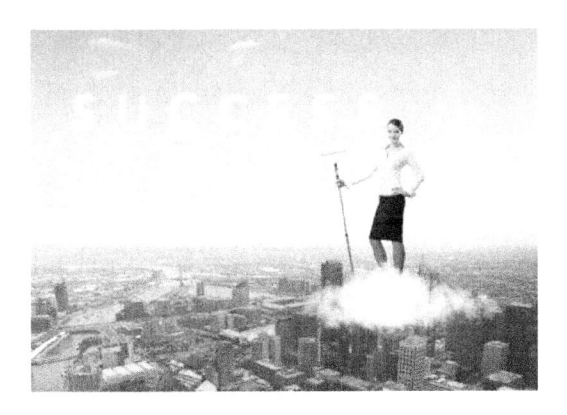

Oh what tangled webs we weave! Unfortunately we're conditioned to fail miserably at the diet thing. Often bracing ourselves for sure failure when still trying to follow through.

There's usually no problem dropping the weight initially. The problems arise with the maintenance end of the deal.

**Most diets are WAY TOO extreme in nature.**

Making it all but impossible to survive the rest of your life drinking just liquids, for example.

With your head working in realistic mode and incorporating the basic **CONCEPT** of the Fast Metabolism Diet, you **WILL** succeed. Don't look at everything through a microscope. Open your mind, and within reason, figure out what does or doesn't work for you.

Use what works and ask questions when something doesn't make sense.

**UNDERSTAND** how and why you're making specific changes, and make them happen.

**NO EXCUSES!**

You're in charge of your life and **YOU** choose whether or not you're going to continue to sabotage yourself by looking for the things that don't work, which of course are everywhere, or not.

It's time for you to decide whether or not you're going to get productive and figure out how you can get happy with your body. A positive decision would mean sticking with the Fast Metabolism Diet concept **LONG-TERM**.

Most people use this concept once or twice a year for about a month, to reach their initial weight loss goals. It's completely up to you. It depends on your wanted results, life situation, preferences, tolerance levels, and desires.

**Here are a few fantastic tips to help you maintain yourself AFTER you've reached the finish line!**

**\*Steer clear of all the processed crap out there.** If you don't know what's in the food you're eating or can't pronounce the ingredient, **DO NOT SWALLOW IT DOWN!**

**\*Stay away mostly from caffeine, alcohol, sugars, soy, and corn**. Of course there will be celebration times, but even then, keep your pants on please!

**\*Go organic when possible.**

**\*Eat IMMEDIATELY upon exiting bed.**

**\*Stick to your meal eating pattern!** -5 mini-meals a day.

**\*Plan your eating ahead, particularly when dining out!**

**\*Cook as much as you can for yourself and freeze for an endless supply.**

**\*Keep drinking water.** Six to eight glasses a day, or at least half your body weight (replace pounds with ounces) EVERY day.

*My Thoughts...*

*Nobody sets out in life to fail. You don't trip and fall on purpose while receiving an award on*

*Stage. Nor do you purposely mark the wrong answers down on a test just to fail.*

*You're looking to change your eating habits because you **want** to look and feel better. This includes losing pesky fat.*

*Having a plan to help sustain your hard work is critical to making your changes stick.*

# Final Thoughts

Life sure would be boring if we were all perfect! If you were happy with your weight, sexy muscles, beautiful eyes, perfect nose, and luscious full lips, you'd get tired of yourself. These physical attributes are what people often believe don't matter.

I'll argue this point because if how you look didn't matter then you wouldn't give a crap.

And you definitely wouldn't be reading any of my diet books!

**Your mental and physical conditions are interconnected.**

If you want to feel good you need to look good. It's what **YOU** think that matters, regardless of the fact we let societal pressures influence our thoughts, feelings, and actions every single day.

Let's deal with the reality here. You want to lose some weight fast before you lose your nerve, in the hopes of bettering yourself as a whole.

The **Fast Metabolism Diet Concept** is an excellent strategy to get you started.

Now that you've read through and understand what metabolism is all about and how you can change your daily actions to do something to improve **YOUR** own, it's time for you to decide what SPECIFIC changes you're going to make in order to get your head and body feel happy and skinny healthy!

Until you physically try out a new concept you don't know how effective it will be. Even if your focus doesn't work **EXACTLY** as planned, so what?

Alter it, try a different approach, or just skip to a new concept altogether.

The important point is not to get discouraged, and **NEVER** ever in a million years give up. If you're a quitter than I can tell you right now you're going to fail miserably.

The only focus I see missing in this eating strategy is exercise.

This concept does mention that exercising triggers and boosts metabolism. But it doesn't **show** you how to get it. Ultimately you need to exercise your body regularly each day. This means doing cardiovascular and muscle-building exercises religiously for up to an hour, 5-6 days a week.

**CIP – CATHY'S IMPORTANT POINT - IF YOU WANT TO LOSE WEIGHT AND KEEP IT OFF YOU MUST EAT NUTRITIOUSLY AND EXERCISE REGULARLY FOR THE REST OF YOUR LIFE**!

You can like it or lump it but it takes hard work to look and feel good. No excuses! It's **YOUR** choice!

It takes time, patience, and a whole lot of **commitment and determination** to get healthy and happy. An exciting challenge indeed.

**Please tell me you're interested!**

*Last Thoughts...*

**\*THANK-YOU** for reading my masterpiece. I hope you learned a little something, or at least got a few smiles.

\*I would appreciate a millisecond or three of your time for a quick review, to help me build my masterful book empire higher.

\*Whatever you do, don't forget to smile, and of course, check out my website for more of my e-Book masterpieces:

www.flawlesscreativewriting.com

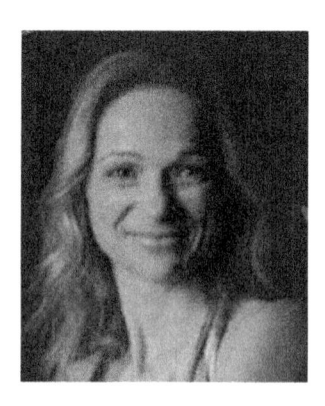

Cathy☺

Printed in Great Britain
by Amazon